THE BEST SALADS AND SIDE DISHES OF ITALIAN VEGETARIAN CUISINE

2021/22

A Concentrate Of Recipes And New Culinary Ideas On Italian Vegetarian Cuisine, The New Recipes Of The Tastiest And Freshest Salads Including Side Dishes That Will Allow You To Start A Healthy Diet And Lose Weight In A Balanced But Steady Way.

Alberto Garofano

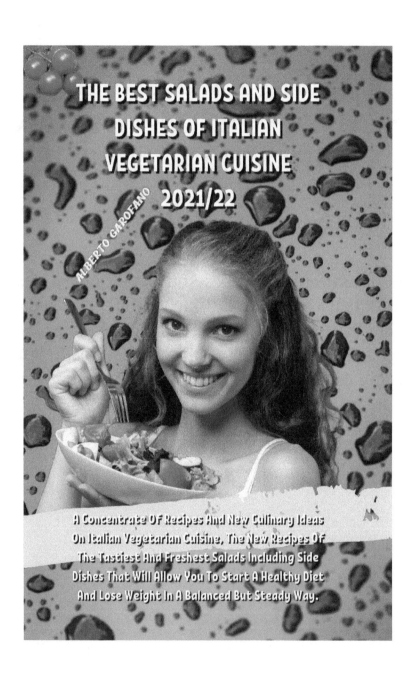

THE BEST SALADS AND SIDE DISHES OF ITALIAN VEGETARIAN CUISINE 2021/22

ALBERTO GAROFANO

A Concentrate Of Recipes And New Culinary Ideas On Italian Vegetarian Cuisine, The New Recipes Of The Tastiest And Freshest Salads Including Side Dishes That Will Allow You To Start A Healthy Diet And Lose Weight In A Balanced But Steady Way.

Table Of Contents

INTRODUCTION 12

CLASSIC EGG SALAD 20

GREEK SALAD 22

POTATO SALAD 24

COLD SLAW 27

CARROT SALAD 29

COLD PASTA SALAD 32

CUCUMBER SALAD WITH SOUR CREAM...............34

TUNA SALAD 37

RICE SALAD 40

HEATED COLESLAW 42

COLORFUL WURSTSALAT 45

MIXED SALAD 47

CUCUMBER SALAD 50

RED BEET SALAD WITH HORSERADISH 52

WALDORF SALAD 55

KOHLRABI SALAD WITH APPLES 58

PAK CHOI SALAD 60

TOMATO SALAD 62

CAESAR SALAD 64

CLASSIC CUCUMBER SALAD 66

VITAL SALAD 68

ICEBERG LETTUCE WITH YOGURT 70

MOZZARELLA ON TOMATO CAPRESE 73

RADISH SALAD 75

COLESLAW.. 76

TOMATO SALAD WITH ONIONS 78

HOUSE STYLE PASTA SALAD... 80

OLIVIER SALAD 82

POTATO SALAD WITH MAYONNAISE 84

ZUCCHINI SALAD... 86

AMERICAN DRESSING 88

SHRIMP COCKTAIL 91

CAESAR DRESSING... 93

BEETROOT SALAD 95

MARINADE FOR POTATO SALAD 97

ASPARAGUS SALAD.. 99

APPLE CELERY SALAD 101

PEPPER SALAD... 104

PASTA SALAD.. 106

FETA AND MELON SALAD... 108

FRENCH DRESSING 110

TZATZIKI 113

TOMATO AND AVOCADO SALAD..115

SHRIMP SALAD 117

POTATO SALAD WITH YOGURT 119

LENTIL SALAD WITH FETA..122

TUNA SALAD WITH RICE...124

CELERY SALAD 126

QUINOA SALAD WITH AVOCADO..128

MEDITERRANEAN PASTA SALAD WITH OLIVE DRESSING...131

CONCLUSIONS 135

The information in the following pages is broadly considered a truthful and accurate account of facts and as such, any inattention, use, or misuse of the information in question by the reader will render any resulting actions solely under their purview. There are no scenarios in which the publisher or the original author of this work can be in any fashion deemed liable for any hardship or damages that may befall them after undertaking information described herein.

Additionally, the information in the following pages is intended only for informational purposes and should thus be thought of as universal. As befitting its nature, it is presented without assurance regarding its prolonged validity or interim quality. Trademarks that are mentioned are done without written consent and can in no way be considered an endorsement from the trademark holder.

☆ *55% OFF for BookStore NOW at $ 30,95 instead of $ 41,95!* ☆

A Concentrate Of Recipes And New Culinary Ideas

On Italian Vegetarian Cuisine, The New Recipes Of

The Tastiest And Freshest Salads Including Side

Dishes That Will Allow You To Start A Healthy Diet

And Lose Weight In A Balanced But Steady Way.

Buy is NOW and let your Customers get addicted to this amazing book!

INTRODUCTION

The vegetarian diet in Italy is spreading widely both for the ease with which vegetables are found in the markets and because they have always been present in the Mediterranean diet. Furthermore, in recent years, with the progressive increase of the world population and the continuous exploitation of the earth's resources, feeding models are being enhanced that have a low environmental impact and can be used for a long time. From these assumptions, diets are born that partially or completely avoid foods of animal origin: the vegetarian diet that does not involve the consumption of meat and fish, molluscs and crustaceans, but allows, in different ways, the consumption of eggs. And dairy products; the vegan diet which, on the other hand, eliminates all products of animal origin.

Following the indications contained in the Guidelines for healthy eating, the vegetarian diet can be formulated to meet the needs of a healthy adult:

- Eat more portions of vegetables and fresh fruit every day
- Increase the consumption of legumes , both fresh and dried
- regularly consume bread, pasta, rice and other cereals , preferably wholemeal
- Eat moderate amounts of fats and oils used for seasoning and cooking. Above all, limit fats of

animal origin (butter, lard, lard, cream, etc.) to season foods and prefer fats of vegetable origin: extra virgin olive oil and seed oils, preferably raw

- Consume eggs and milk that contain good organic quality proteins. If you drink a lot of milk, preferably choose the skim or semi-skim one which, however, maintains its calcium and vitamin content
- Eat cheeses in moderate quantities because in addition to proteins they contain high amounts of fat. For this reason it is advisable to choose the leaner ones, or eat smaller portions
- Limit foods rich in fat, salt and sugar such as creams, chocolate, chips, biscuits, sweets, ice cream, cakes and puddings to special occasions

The Elements That Cannot Be Missing In A Vegetarian Diet

The first thing to watch out for is to follow a diet that is as varied as possible. Some nutrients are present in small amounts in vegetables, or are less easily absorbed by the body than those from meat or fish. However, most vegetarians generally do not have ailments due to nutrient deficiencies if they take care to include certain foods in their diet:

- Legumes combined with cereals, to ensure the availability, in addition to significant quantities of starch and fiber, of essential nutrients characteristic of meat, fish and eggs, such as iron, proteins of good biological quality, micronutrients

- Foods obtained from wholemeal flours (and not with the simple addition of bran or other fibers) which, in addition to starch and fiber, contain good amounts of calcium, iron and B vitamins

If not formulated correctly, the vegetarian diet can be deficient in essential nutrients. Those who follow it need to make sure they get sufficient amounts of iron and vitamin B12 with their food.

Plant Sources Of Iron

Vegetarians may have less iron in their body stores than people who also eat meat. It is therefore important to know the foods, suitable for vegetarians, which contain a good amount of iron:

- Eggs
- Legumes (especially lentils)
- Dried fruit
- Pumpkin seeds
- Vegetables (especially dark green ones)
- Whole grain bread
- Plant Sources of Vitamin B12

Vitamin B12 is needed for growth, cell repair, and overall health. It is found, in nature, only in products of animal origin such as, for example, meat, fish, shellfish, eggs and dairy products. If you eat these foods regularly, you are likely to be getting enough of them. However, if you only eat small amounts of foods of animal origin, or if you avoid them altogether, it is important to include certain sources of vitamin B12 in your diet:

- Milk
- Cheese
- Eggs

If the amount of vitamin B12 introduced in the diet is insufficient to meet the body's needs, it is advisable to also use foods in which it is added (fortified foods) such as:

- Fortified breakfast cereals
- Fortified soy products
- Plant sources of omega-3

The omega-3 fatty acids are found mainly in oily fish, fresh tuna and salmon. Plant sources of omega-3 fatty acids include:

- Flax seed
- Rapeseed oil
- Soybean oil and soy-based foods (such as tofu)
- Nuts

Being Vegetarian In Particular Conditions

Those who wish to follow a vegetarian diet during childhood, pregnancy, advanced age or in conjunction with illnesses, must rely on a doctor or nutritionist, because in such conditions their needs for nutrients may vary. For example, during pregnancy and breastfeeding, women following a vegetarian diet need to ensure that the amounts of vitamins and minerals in their diet are sufficient to ensure that their baby can grow healthily. While growing up, the parent must ensure that the child eats a very varied diet to meet the nutritional needs he needs.

START

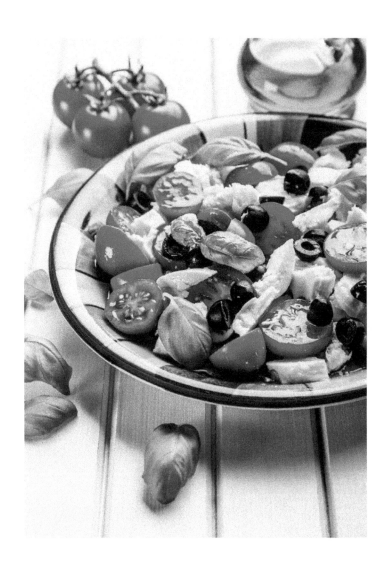

CLASSIC EGG SALAD

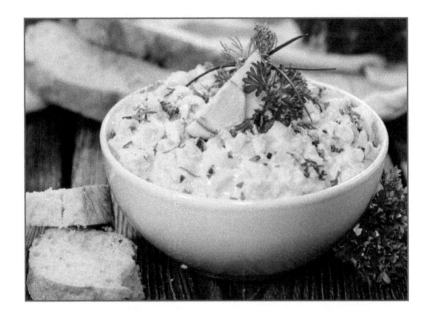

Servings:4

INGREDIENTS

- 8 Pc Eggs
- 2 Tbsp mayonnaise
- 2 Tbsp sour cream
- 0.5 TL mustard
- 1 Tbsp vinegar
- 1 prize salt
- 1 prize Pepper from the grinder)

PREPARATION

1. For the classic egg salad, first boil the eggs hard in a saucepan with water for around 10 minutes.
2. Then lift it out of the pot and rinse in cold water, peel and chop into small pieces.
3. Now mix the mayonnaise with salt, pepper, vinegar and sour cream well in a bowl.
4. Mix in the eggs and let them steep in the refrigerator for three hours.
5. After steeping in the refrigerator, season the salad again with salt, pepper and possibly a little mustard.

GREEK SALAD

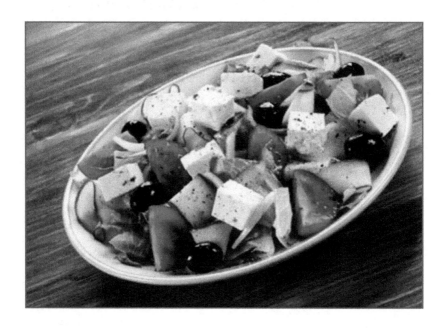

Servings:4

INGREDIENTS

- 1 Pc small onion
- 1 prize Seasoned Salt
- 4 Pc Olives
- 3 Tbsp olive oil
- 1 Pc Cucumber
- 50 G Sheep cheese
- 2 Pc tomatoes

for the vinaigrette

- 2 TL salt
- 1 TL sugar
- 1 shot vinegar
- 200 ml water

PREPARATION

1. Wash tomatoes and cut into wedges.
2. Wash the cucumber and cut into long thin strips.
3. Cut the onion into thin rings and mix with the cut vegetables.
4. Pour 3 tablespoons of olive oil over it, as well as the mixed vinaigrette, then stir everything together and season with herb salt.
5. Now you can add the pitted olives and the crushed sheep's cheese to the salad.

POTATO SALAD

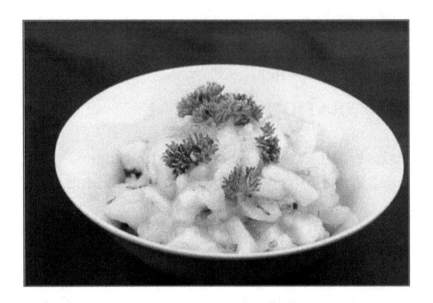

Servings:4

INGREDIENTS

- 400 G Potato (greasy)
- 100 G Onions (finely chopped)
- for the marinade
- 1 Tbsp Dijon mustard
- 5 Tbsp Corn oil
- 120 ml Beef soup (warm)
- 5 Tbsp Hesperide vinegar
- 1 TL Salt (deleted)

- 2 TL Sugar (deleted)
- 80 ml Water (lukewarm)
-

PREPARATION

1. Cook the potatoes with their skins in salted water for approx. 40 minutes until firm to the bite, drain, rinse with cold water, peel while still warm and cut into slices.
2. Then peel and finely chop the onion and add to the potato slices.
3. Mix all marinade ingredients well in a bowl, pour over the still lukewarm potatoes and leave to stand for about 30 minutes.

COLD SLAW

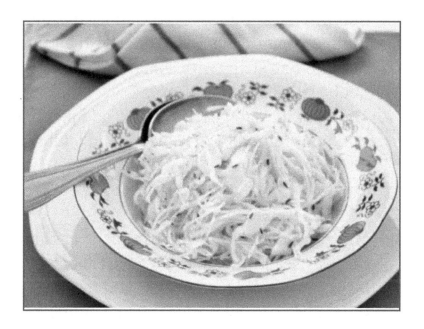

Servings:6

INGREDIENTS

- 1 kpf White cabbage
- 3 Tbsp salt
- 2 TL pepper
- 150 ml Mineral water
- for the marinade
- 6 Tbsp oil
- 4 Tbsp Herb vinegar
- 1 Tbsp sugar
- 1 TL Caraway seed

PREPARATION

1. Remove the outer leaves from the cabbage head, cut out the stalk and quarter the cabbage. Cut into fine strips with a sharp knife or grate finely with a kitchen slicer.
2. Then put the cabbage in a bowl, add plenty of salt, pour mineral water over it and let it steep for about 30 minutes.
3. Then pour off the excess water and squeeze out the herb well with your hands.
4. Mix a marinade from vinegar, oil, sugar and caraway seeds and pour over the cabbage. Season with plenty of pepper and mix well.
5. Cover the coleslaw and let it steep in the refrigerator for a few hours.

CARROT SALAD

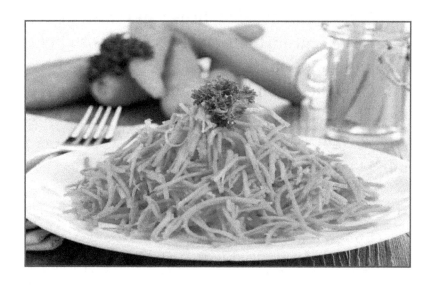

Servings:4

INGREDIENTS

- 400 G Carrots
- 1 TL honey
- 0.5 Pc Lemon, juice

For the vinaigrette

- 1 shot oil
- 100 ml water
- 0.5 TL salt
- 1 shot Vinegar (light, of your choice)

PREPARATION

1. For the carrot salad, brush and wash the carrots, grate them finely, season with honey and lemon juice.
2. Only the oil on top and the vinaigrette.
3. The vinaigrette is made from water, salt and vinegar.
4. Let stand for at least 30 minutes.

COLD PASTA SALAD

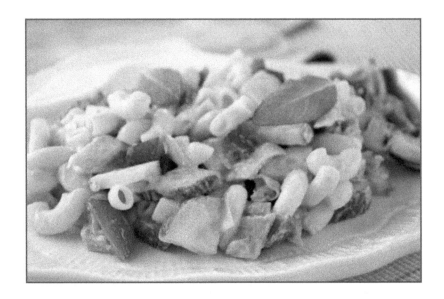

Servings:4

INGREDIENTS

- 2 Pc Paprika (colored)
- 3 Pc tomatoes
- 1 Pc cucumber
- 400 G ham
- 400 G Pasta
- 0.5 cups yogurt
- 0.5 cups sour cream
- 0.5 TL salt
- 1 prize Pepper from the grinder)

- 1 shot vinegar
-

PREPARATION

1. For the cold pasta salad, first cook the pasta in a pan with salted water until it is firm to the bite, then strain and refrigerate.
2. In the meantime, wash, clean and chop the tomatoes, peppers and cucumbers.
3. Also cut the ham into thin strips.
4. Put the vegetables, pasta and ham in a bowl.
5. Mix the sour cream, yoghurt, salt, pepper and vinegar into a dressing and pour over the salad. Mix everything well.

CUCUMBER SALAD WITH SOUR CREAM

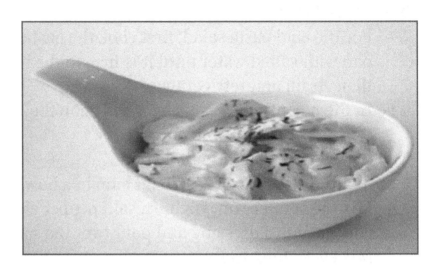

Servings:4

INGREDIENTS

- 2 Pc Cucumbers
- 1 cups sour cream
- 1 Tbsp oil
- 4 Tbsp Balsamic vinegar
- 1 Pc onion
- 2 Pc Garlic cloves
- 1 Federation dill
- 1 prize salt

PREPARATION

1. Slice the peeled cucumber, place in a bowl, season with salt and leave to stand for about 20 minutes.
2. Then squeeze out the cucumber well and place in a salad bowl.
3. Finely chop the dill and chop the peeled garlic and onion.
4. For the dressing, mix the sour cream, vinegar, oil, onions, garlic and dill and pour over the cucumber.
5. Stir and let steep for about 10 minutes.

TUNA SALAD

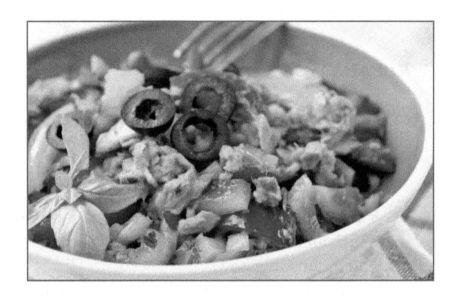

Servings:2

INGREDIENTS

- 1 Can tuna
- 1 Pc Red peppers
- 1 Pc Green peppers
- 200 G Cocktail tomatoes
- 0.5 Pc Onion red
- 0.5 Federation parsley

For the dressing
- 2 Tbsp Lemon juice
- 3 Tbsp olive oil

- 1 prize salt
- 1 prize pepper
- 1 shot water
-

PREPARATION

1. First wash, core and cut the bell peppers into thin slices.
2. Wash tomatoes and cut in half.
3. Peel the onion and cut into thin rings.
4. Then strain the tuna, divide the meat apart with a fork and mix well with the peppers, tomatoes and onions in a bowl.
5. For the dressing 1 mix well a little water, lemon juice, oil, salt and pepper and marinate the salad with it.
6. Finally, wash the parsley, chop it finely and sprinkle it over the tuna salad.

RICE SALAD

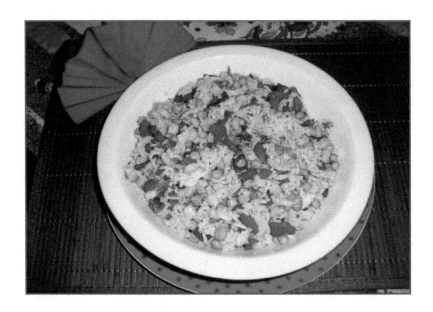

Servings:6

INGREDIENTS

- 300 G Long grain rice
- 80 G Peas, fresh or frozen
- 3 Pc Spring onions, in rings
- 1 Pc green peppers, finely diced
- 1 Pc red peppers, finely diced
- 300 G Canned corn kernels
- 15   G Mint, crushed

For the dressing

- 1 Pc Clove of garlic (crushed)
- 125 ml Olive oil (native)
- 2 Tbsp Lemon juice
- 1 TL sugar
- 1 prize pepper
- 1 prize salt
-

PREPARATION

1. For the rice salad, bring the water to the boil in a large saucepan and stir in the rice.
2. Bring to the boil and simmer for 12-15 minutes, until the rice is firm to the bite.
3. Drain and let cool.
4. Boil the peas for approx. 2 minutes in a small saucepan with boiling water. Rinse under cold water and drain well.
5. For the dressing, mix the oil, lemon juice, garlic and sugar in a small mixing bowl and whisk well. Season to taste with salt and freshly ground black pepper.
6. Put the rice, peas, spring onions, bell pepper, corn, and mint in a large bowl. Add the dressing and mix well.
7. Cover and put in the fridge for 1 hour.
8. Then transfer to a salad bowl.

HEATED COLESLAW

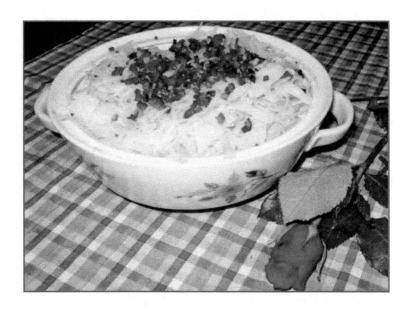

Servings: 2

INGREDIENTS

- 1 shot vinegar
- 100 G bacon
- 1 kpf White cabbage
- 1 Tbsp sugar
- 1 Pc onion
- 1 prize Caraway seed
- 1 prize pepper
- 1 prize salt

PREPARATION

1. For the coleslaw, remove the stalk from the cabbage and cut into fine noodles.
2. Then fry the bacon in a saucepan, sprinkle the sugar over it and let it caramelize a little.
3. Set aside some pieces of bacon for decoration.
4. Deglaze with vinegar and finally add the cabbage.
5. Mix everything well, add the spices.
6. Pour water on until the herb is just covered. Then steam until soft.
7. Stir occasionally.
8. Put the salad in a bowl, add a few pieces of bacon on top as a decoration and serve.

COLORFUL WURSTSALAT

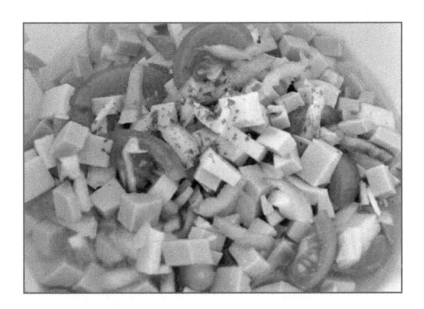

Servings:2

INGREDIENTS

- 3 Tbsp Apple Cider Vinegar
- 1 Tbsp Oil (preferably pumpkin seed oil)
- 1 TL Estragon mustard
- 2 Pc Geezer
- 1 Pc Medium onion
- 1 Pc Paprika (yellow)
- 2 Pc tomatoes
- 2 Pc Eggs (hard-boiled)

- 1 Pc Paprika (green)
- 1 Tbsp chives
- 1 prize sugar
- 1 prize pepper
- 1 prize salt
-

PREPARATION

1. The crackers are cut into as thin slices as possible.
2. Now add the diced onion, the peppers cut into strips and the tomatoes cut into wedges.
3. Season with salt, pepper and sugar.
4. Finally add the apple cider vinegar and, depending on the acidity of the vinegar, some water and 1 teaspoon of tarragon, mix well.
5. Finally add the oil, mix again and decorate with freshly chopped chives and hard-boiled eggs (cut into slices or wedges).

MIXED SALAD

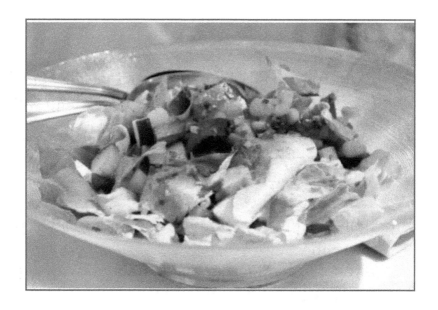

Servings:4

INGREDIENTS

- 1 kpf green salad
- 1 Pc Cucumber
- 4 Pc tomatoes
- 2 Pc paprika
- 1 Can Corn
- 3 Tbsp oil
- 6 Tbsp vinegar
- 1 prize salt
- 1 prize pepper

- 1 Tbsp mustard
-

PREPARATION

1. Remove the stalk from the green lettuce, pluck the leaves off individually and wash them well. Wash the cucumber, tomatoes and peppers.
2. Tear the lettuce leaves into bite-sized pieces. Halve the cucumber lengthways and dice.
3. Cut the tomatoes into small pieces.
4. Remove the core from the pepper and also cut into cubes.
5. Put the vegetables in a large bowl, season with salt and stir well.
6. Drain the canned corn in a colander and add to the bowl.
7. Mix a dressing from oil, vinegar, mustard, salt and pepper.
8. Pour over the salad, stir well and let stand for a few minutes.

CUCUMBER SALAD

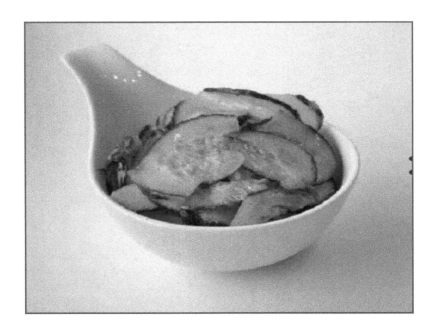

Servings:3

INGREDIENTS

- 1 Pc Cucumber
- 0.5 TL salt
- 1 prize Garlic pepper
- 3 Tbsp Apple Cider Vinegar
- 3 Tbsp Sunflower oil
- 1 Tbsp sugar

PREPARATION

1. Wash the cucumber, cut off the ends and cut into thin slices or grate.
2. Mix the salt into the sliced cucumber and let stand for about a quarter of an hour.
3. Squeeze out the cucumber and throw away the water.
4. Add vinegar, oil, garlic pepper and sugar and stir everything well.

RED BEET SALAD WITH HORSERADISH

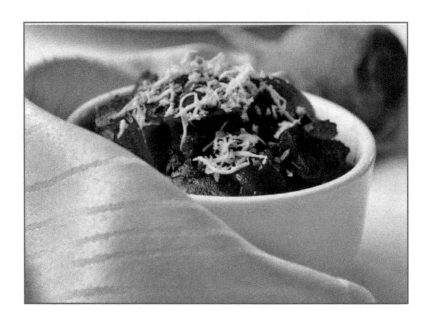

Servings:4

INGREDIENTS

- 0.5 kg Beetroot
- 0.5 Cup vinegar
- 1 Tbsp salt
- 1 Tbsp sugar
- 1 Tbsp Caraway seed
- 3 Tbsp Horseradish (grated)

PREPARATION

1. Cook the beets in a saucepan of water for an hour until they are soft.
2. Then peel and cut into leaves.
3. Bring the vinegar to the boil with a little water, salt and sugar. Sprinkle the caraway seeds over the beets, pour the marinade over them and leave to stand for a few hours. Sprinkle the salad with freshly grated horseradish before serving.

WALDORF SALAD

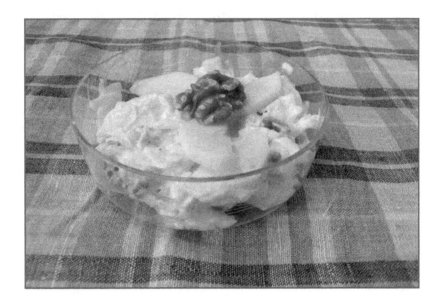

Servings:4

INGREDIENTS

- 4 Pc Apples
- 200 G Walnut kernels
- 1 Pc Celery bulb
- 1 Pc Lemon (juice)
- 100 G Semi-fat mayonnaise
- 125 G sour cream
- 1 Tbsp sugar
- 1 prize pepper
- 1 prize salt

PREPARATION

1. Clean, peel, wash, quarter and briefly boil over the celery.
2. Then coarsely grate the cooked celery.
3. Peel, quarter, core and slice apples.
4. Roughly chop the nuts and mix well with the lemon juice, salt, sugar and pepper.
5. Finally, fold in mayonnaise and sour cream.
6. Then put the whole mixture in a cool place.

KOHLRABI SALAD WITH APPLES

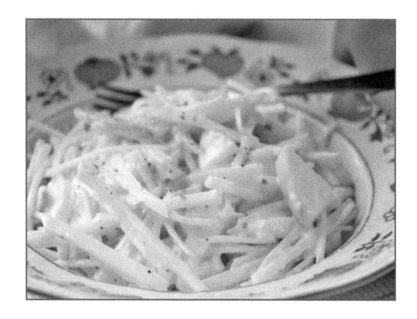

Servings:4

INGREDIENTS

- 0.5 cups sour cream
- 1 Pc onion
- 0.5 Federation parsley
- 1 Pc Lemons (juice)
- 1 Tbsp honey
- 800 G Kohlrabi
- 2 Pc Apples
- 1 prize pepper
- 1 prize salt

PREPARATION

1. Peel the apples and kohlrabi and grate finely. Peel onions and cut them into fine pieces.
2. Wash, drain and chop the parsley.
3. Mix lemon juice, honey, salt, pepper and sour cream into a dressing.
4. Pour the sauce over the salad and mix well.

PAK CHOI SALAD

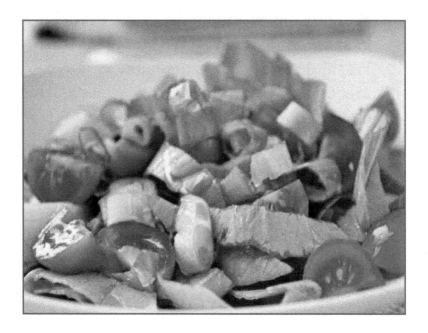

Servings: 2

INGREDIENTS

- 4 Stg Pak choi
- 2 Pc tomatoes
- 3 Pc Spring onion
- 3 Pc hot peppers
- 1 Tbsp Balsamic vinegar (white)
- 1 prize salt
- 1 prize pepper
- 1 prize sugar
- 3 Tbsp Sunflower oil

- 1 Tbsp sesame oil

PREPARATION

1. For the pak choi salad, first cut the stalks of the pak choi into cubes about one centimeter and the leaves into pieces of the appropriate size. Wash and core the tomatoes and cut them into one-centimeter pieces.
2. Wash the spring onions and peppers and cut into rings.
3. Now mix the vinegar, salt, pepper and sugar together. Vigorously knock in the sunflower oil with a fork.
4. Then briefly stir in the sesame oil. Mix the salad ingredients together.
5. Pour the marinade over it and fold in briefly.

TOMATO SALAD

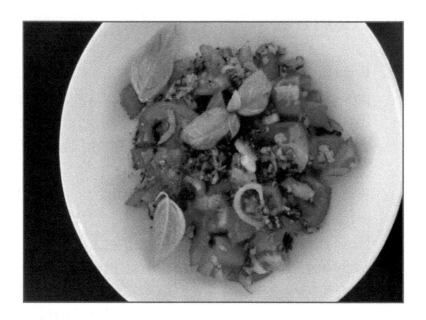

Servings:1

INGREDIENTS

- 1 Tbsp basil
- 3 Tbsp olive oil
- 1 prize salt
- 3 Pc tomatoes
- 1 Pc onion
- 1 shot Lemon juice
- 1 shot vinegar
- 1 prize sugar

PREPARATION

1. Cut tomatoes into slices (or wedges).
2. Peel the onion, cut into cubes and add to the tomatoes with the finely chopped basil.
3. Then add the olive oil, a dash of vinegar, lemon juice and a pinch of sugar, mix well and season with salt.

CAESAR SALAD

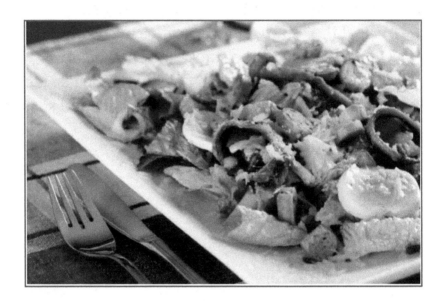

Servings:4

INGREDIENTS

- 1 Pc Baguette, for the croutons
- 2 Tbsp Olive oil, for the croutons
- 1 Pc Garlic clove, for the croutons
- 4 Pc Anchovy fillets
- 1 Pc Garlic cloves
- 20 G Freshly grated parmesan
- 1 Tbsp Red wine vinegar
- 1 TL hot mustard
- 80 ml olive oil

- 1 kpf Romaine lettuce
- 1 prize pepper
- 2 Pc Egg yolk
- 2 Pc onion

PREPARATION

1. For the croutons, cut the baguette into small cubes.
2. Heat the oil in a large pan.
3. Peel and squeeze the garlic clove and stir into the oil. Turn the heat down and add the baguette cubes to the pan. Lightly brown on all sides, stirring constantly.
4. Then let cool on a plate.
5. For the dressing, cut the 2 anchovies into small pieces and roughly chop the garlic cloves.
6. Mix the anchovies, garlic, Parmesan, vinegar, mustard and egg yolks in a tall, narrow vessel with a hand blender. Add the oil in a fine stream, stirring further until a creamy sauce is formed. Season to taste with pepper.
7. Clean and wash romaine lettuce. Pluck the leaves into bite-sized pieces. Cut the anchovy fillet into narrow strips.

CLASSIC CUCUMBER SALAD

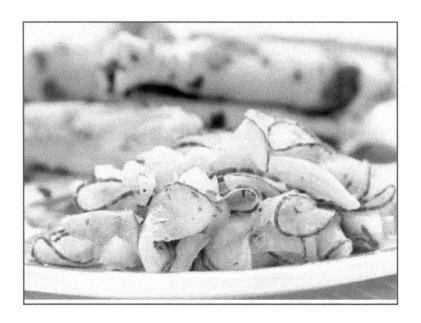

Servings:4

INGREDIENTS

- 2 Pc Cucumber
- 1 Pc onion
- 15 G sugar
- 1 TL salt
- 4 Tbsp oil
- 4 Tbsp vinegar

PREPARATION

1. Wash the cucumber and cut into slices.
2. Peel the onion and cut into rings.
3. Mix all ingredients and season again to taste. Let it steep for 10 minutes.

VITAL SALAD

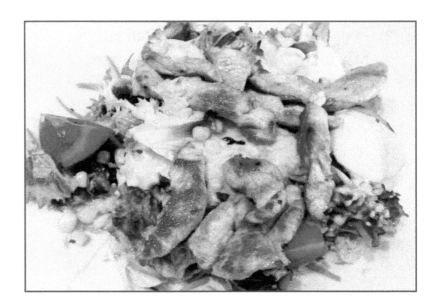

Servings:4

INGREDIENTS

- 1 Can Corn
- 6 Pc Cocktail tomatoes
- 1 Pc endive salad
- 2 Pc carrot
- 1 Pc Cucumber
- 1 kg Turkey meat
- 1 Tbsp Paprika powder
- 1 shot olive oil

Ingredients for the dressing

- 1 shot olive oil
- 4 Tbsp yogurt
- 1 TL mustard
- 2 Tbsp Balsamic vinegar

PREPARATION

1. Wash and pick the lettuce.
2. Grate the carrot into fine strips, cut the cucumber into slices.
3. Quarter the tomatoes and take the corn out of the tin and rinse with cold water.
4. Mix the dressing made from yogurt, olive oil, mustard and balsamic vinegar in a bowl and let it steep. (approx. 20-30 min.)
5. Meanwhile, cut the meat into strips, season with salt and pepper and season with a pinch of red paprika powder.
6. Heat the olive oil in a pan and fry the meat in it for a few minutes.
7. Arrange the lettuce leaves on plates, place the cut vegetables on top and pour the dressing over them.
8. Just put the meat on the salad and serve with white bread.

ICEBERG LETTUCE WITH YOGURT

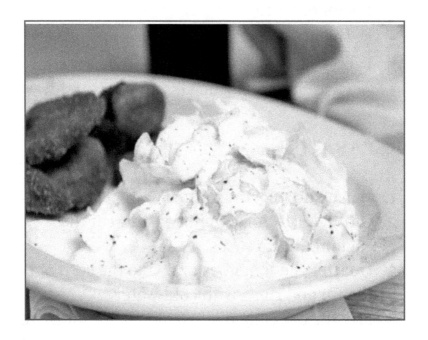

Servings:4

INGREDIENTS

- 1 cups yogurt
- 1 Pc Iceberg lettuce
- 2 Tbsp Lemon juice
- 2 Tbsp olive oil
- 1 prize sugar
- 1 prize pepper
- 1 prize salt

PREPARATION

1. Divide the lettuce, pluck it into bite-sized pieces and then wash it well. Drain.
2. For the dressing, mix the remaining ingredients well in a bowl.
3. Mix the dressing with the salad well.

MOZZARELLA ON TOMATO CAPRESE

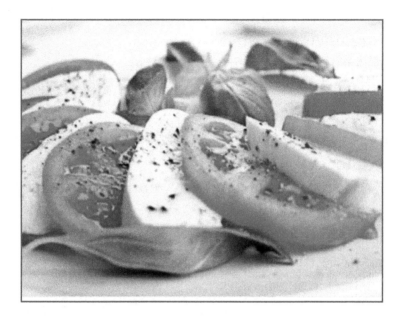

Servings:4

INGREDIENTS

- 1 shot Balsamic vinegar
- 1 Federation basil
- 3 Pc clove of garlic
- 300 G Mozzarella
- 4 Tbsp olive oil
- 4 Pc ripe beefsteak tomatoes
- 1 prize pepper
- 1 prize salt

PREPARATION

1. Wash the tomatoes and cut them into slices, removing the stalks.
2. Arrange on a platter or a large plate.
3. Peel and finely chop the garlic and sprinkle over the tomatoes.
4. Salt, pepper and drizzle with 2 tablespoons of oil.
5. Wash the basil, shake dry and cut the leaves into fine strips.
6. Drain the mozzarella well and cut into slices. Cover the tomato slices with the mozzarella slices.
7. Drizzle with the remaining olive oil and serve sprinkled with the basil.
8. Suffice it with balsamic vinegar so that everyone can drizzle a little over the mozzarella as they wish.

RADISH SALAD

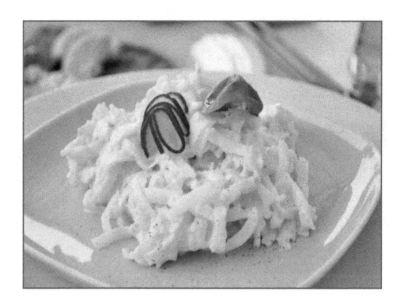

Servings:4

INGREDIENTS

- 500 G radish
- 250 ml sour cream
- 2 Tbsp vinegar
- 1 TL salt

PREPARATION

1. The radish must be roughly grated and then mixed with the vinegar, cream and salt.

COLESLAW

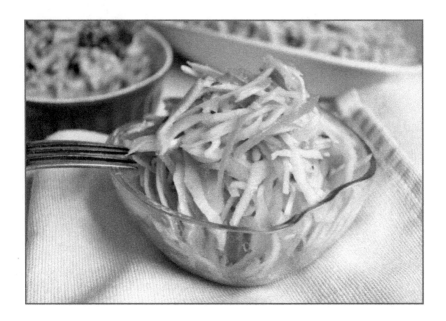

Servings:4

INGREDIENTS

- 350 G White cabbage
- 3 Pc Carrots
- 1 TL salt
- 1 prize pepper
- 1 TL Caraway seed

Ingredients for the marinade
- 3 Tbsp oil
- 2 Tbsp vinegar
- 1 prize sugar

- 1 prize salt
- 1 TL Mustard medium hot
-

PREPARATION

2. Clean and slice the white cabbage.
3. Wash in a colander and drain. Peel the carrots and slice into pens.
4. Mix the cabbage and carrots, season with salt and stir well. Let it steep for 1 hour.
5. Mix the oil, vinegar, mustard, sugar, pepper and salt to a marinade.
6. Squeeze out the cabbage and carrots, discard the resulting liquid.
7. Pour the marinade over the cabbage and carrots, mix well and sprinkle with caraway seeds.
8. Let it steep for another 0.5 hour.

TOMATO SALAD WITH ONIONS

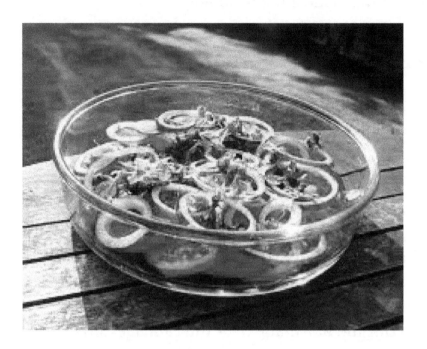

Servings:4

INGREDIENTS

- 7 Tbsp olive oil
- 4 Tbsp vinegar
- 1 prize salt
- 1 Pc onion
- 10 Pc tomatoes

PREPARATION

1. For the tomato salad with onions, first wash the tomatoes, pat dry, remove the stalk and cut into slices.
2. Now peel the onion and cut into rings.
3. Put in a bowl and mix with salt, vinegar and oil. Add the tomato slices and fold in carefully.

HOUSE STYLE PASTA SALAD

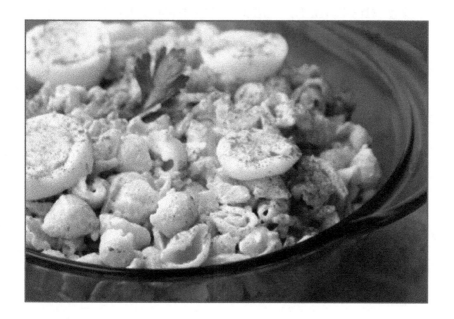

Servings:4

INGREDIENTS

- 500 G Pasta
- 1 Can Peas
- 1 Can Mushrooms
- 1 Pc Peppers (red or yellow)
- 4 Pc Eggs
- 3 Pc pickled cucumbers
- 1cups yogurt
- 3 Tbsp Cucumber water (from the pickles)
- 1 cups Creme Fresh

- 1 prize pepper
- 1 prize salt
-

PREPARATION

1. Cook the pasta in lightly salted water until al dente.
2. Hard boil eggs.
3. Rinse the pasta and eggs with cold water and place in a large bowl.
4. Add the peas and mushrooms.
5. Cut the cucumber into thin slices. Finely dice the paprika.
6. Add both to the rest and mix everything well.
7. Mix the yoghurt with Creme Fresh and two to three tablespoons of cucumber water in an extra container.
8. Season to taste with pepper and salt.
9. Then gradually mix the sauce into the rest of the ingredients.

OLIVIER SALAD

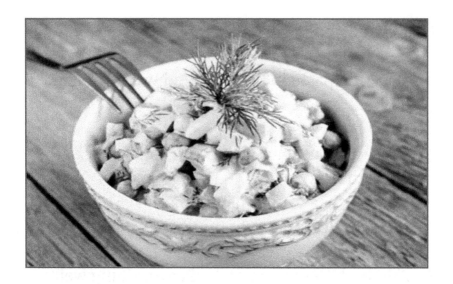

Servings:4
INGREDIENTS
- 300 G Chicken (fried)
- 300 G Potatoes
- 150 G Carrots
- 150 G onion
- 100 G Pickle Guy
- 400 G Peas
- 3 Pc   hard-boiled eggs
- 1 Pc   Apple (sour)
- 150 ml mayonnaise
- 1 prize pepper
- 1 prize salt

PREPARATION

1. For the Olivier salad, first boil the potatoes (with their skin) and carrots in water (approx. 20 minutes).
2. In the meantime, cut the cooked chicken into small pieces.
3. Now boil the eggs (approx. 10 min.), Let them cool, peel and finely chop.
4. Peel onions and cut them into fine pieces.
5. Peel the cooked and slightly cooled potatoes and cut into small cubes.
6. Then peel and core the apple and cut into small cubes.
7. Also cut the pickles into fine cubes or slices.
8. Finally, put all the ingredients in a bowl, drain and add the peas, mix well with the mayonnaise.

POTATO SALAD WITH MAYONNAISE

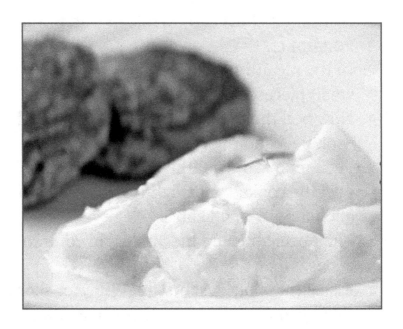

Servings:4

INGREDIENTS

- 600 G Potatoes
- 1 Pc onion
- 200 G mayonnaise
- 3 Tbsp vinegar
- 2 Tbsp sour cream
- 1 TL salt
- 1 prize Pepper from the grinder)

PREPARATION

1. For the potato salad with mayonnaise, first cook the potatoes in a saucepan with salted water until they are soft.
2. Let cool a little, peel and cut into slices. Put in a bowl.
3. In the meantime, peel and finely chop the onion, add to the potatoes.
4. For the dressing, mix together the mayonnaise, vinegar, sour cream, salt and pepper.
5. Pour over the salad and stir gently.

ZUCCHINI SALAD

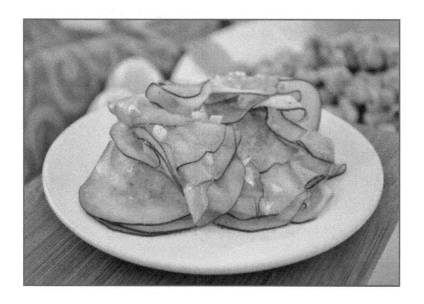

Servings:4

INGREDIENTS

- 1 Pc zucchini
- 3 Pc Garlic cloves
- 3 Tbsp vinegar
- 3 Tbsp oil
- 1 TL salt
- 1 prize pepper

PREPARATION

1. Wash the zucchini and cut lengthways without peeling, remove the stones if necessary.
2. Then slice the zucchini or cut into fine sticks. Peel the garlic and chop in to fine slithers.
3. Mix the vinegar, garlic, oil and the spices in a bowl and add the grated zucchini, mix and refrigerate for about 1 hour.

AMERICAN DRESSING

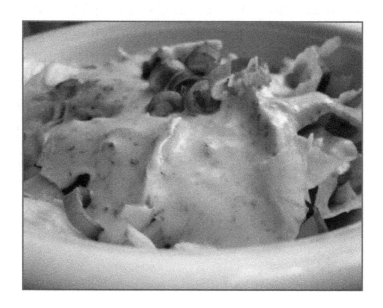

Servings:4

INGREDIENTS

- 0.5 cups Creme fraiche Cheese
- 1 Tbsp freshly chopped herbs
- 1 cups yogurt
- 1 TL Paradeisketchup
- 0.5 TL mustard
- 1 Spr Lemon juice
- 3 Tbsp oil
- 1 prize salt
- 1 prize sugar

PREPARATION

1. Put all ingredients such as crème fraiche, parade ice-cream ketchup, yoghurt, herbal tea, oil, mustard and lemon juice in a bowl and mix well with a mixer.
2. Shake the bowl vigorously and the salad dressing is ready.

SHRIMP COCKTAIL

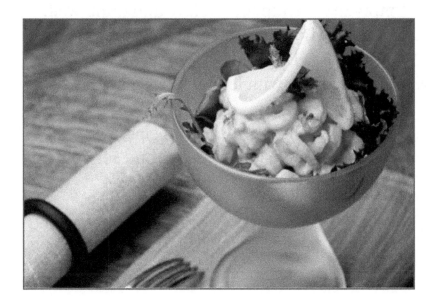

Servings:6

INGREDIENTS

- 2 TL Curry powder
- 300 G mayonnaise
- 1 prize salt
- 1 prize pepper
- 3 Tbsp milk
- 2 Tbsp Peppercorns
- 3 Tbsp Chives, chopped
- 1 Tbsp Lemon juice
- 600 G Shrimp

PREPARATION

1. Empty the shrimp into a sieve and drain well.
2. Mix the shrimp, peppercorns, mayonnaise and milk in a bowl.
3. Season to taste with lemon juice, curry, sugar, salt and pepper.
4. Arrange the shrimp cocktail in glasses, garnish with chives and a lemon wedge and serve immediately.

CAESAR DRESSING

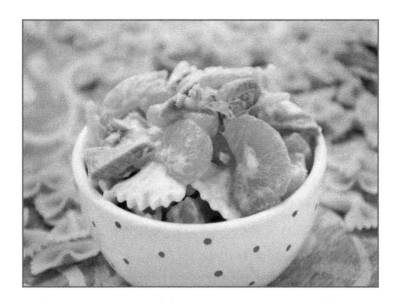

Servings:1

INGREDIENTS

- 4 Tbsp Parmesan
- 1 prize sugar
- 1 prize salt
- 1 prize pepper
- 1 Spr Worcester sauce
- 1 Spr mustard
- 50 ml water
- 2 Pc egg yolk
- 100 ml olive oil

- 1 Spr Lemon juice
- 1 Pc clove of garlic
-

PREPARATION

1. For the Caesar dressing , the garlic must be peeled and finely chopped.
2. Mix the lemon juice, the garlic pieces, the egg yolks and a dash of mustard in a bowl.
3. Now puree some water, a splash of Worcestershire sauce, salt, pepper and a pinch of sugar with the blender.
4. At the end the olive oil is slowly added. Continue to mix the almost finished Caesar dressing well and refine it with the parmesan at the end.

BEETROOT SALAD

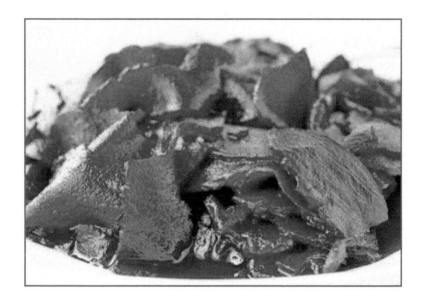

Servings:2

INGREDIENTS

- 2 Pc Beetroot
- 2 Tbsp vinegar
- 1 TL sugar
- 1 TL salt
- 1 TL Caraway seed

PREPARATION

1. For the beetroot salad, wash the beets and cook them in salted water on a low heat for 30 minutes.
2. Rinse the boiled beets with cold water, peel and cut into thin slices.
3. Let the vinegar boil for five minutes with a little water, salt, caraway seeds and sugar, pour over the beets, cover with cling film and let sit in the refrigerator.

MARINADE FOR POTATO SALAD

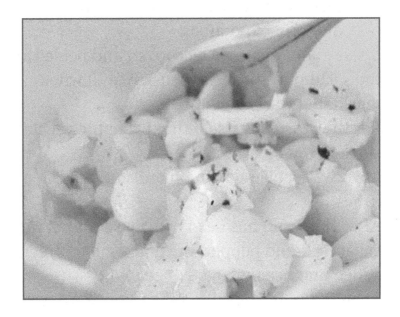

Servings:4

INGREDIENTS

- 50 ml vinegar
- 400 ml Vegetable broth
- 80 ml oil
- 1 Tbsp mustard
- 1 TL sugar
- 1 Pc Onion (red)
- 1 prize salt
- 1 prize pepper

PREPARATION

1. This tasty, hearty marinade is enough for about one kilogram of potatoes.
2. These should already be cooked and peeled and the salad pulls itself particularly well when marinated warm.
3. For the marinade itself, first bring the vegetable stock to the boil.
4. Meanwhile, peel the onion and cut into fine cubes.
5. After the broth has been heavily seasoned with sugar, salt and pepper, the onion cubes are added and briefly boiled once.
6. Then stir in the vinegar, oil and mustard well. Like the potatoes, the marinade should also be fairly warm when the potato salad is marinated. It is best to let it sit for several hours and then enjoy.

ASPARAGUS SALAD

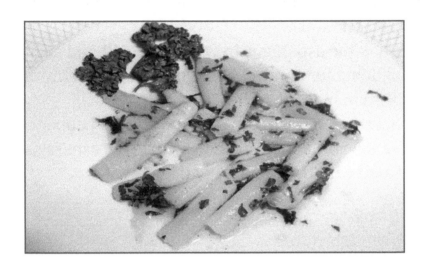

Servings:4

INGREDIENTS

- 1 shot vinegar
- 1 TL olive oil
- 1 Federation parsley
- 1 kg White asparagus (peeled)
- 1 TL sugar
- 0.5 Tbsp Butter to pan
- 1 prize pepper
- 1 prize salt

PREPARATION

1. Cut off the ends of the asparagus approx. 1 cm, peel and wash.
2. Cook the asparagus in water with salt and sugar al dente for approx. 12-15 minutes, then strain. Toss in butter.
3. Season the warm asparagus with salt, pepper, vinegar and olive oil and sprinkle the asparagus salad with the chopped parsley.

APPLE CELERY SALAD

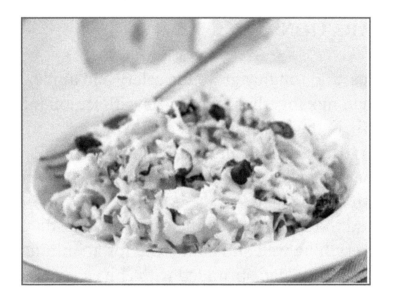

Servings:4

INGREDIENTS

- 350 G celery root
- 1   Pc Apple
- 2 Tbsp Lemon juice
- 2 Tbsp Raisins
- 2 Tbsp chopped hazelnuts
- 150 G yogurt
- 2 Tbsp mayonnaise
- 2 Tbsp vinegar
- 1 prize pepper

- 1 prize chives
- 1 prize salt
-

PREPARATION

1. Peel and roughly grate the celery and apple, then mix together and drizzle with lemon juice.
2. Mix in the hazelnuts and raisins.
3. In the meantime, mix the yoghurt with the mayonnaise, add the vinegar and season with salt and pepper.
4. Add the sauce to the other ingredients, stir everything well and let it steep for 30 minutes.
5. Serve the salad sprinkled with chives.

PEPPER SALAD

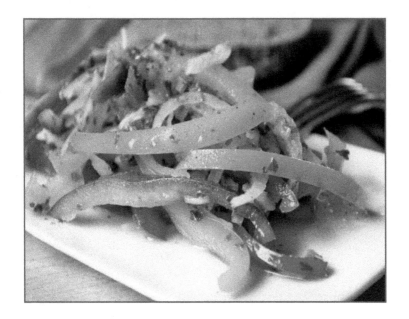

Servings:4

INGREDIENTS

- 4 Pc Paprika (colored)
- 1 Pc Onion (large)
- 5 Tbsp water
- 3 Tbsp oil
- 2 Tbsp vinegar
- 2 Tbsp Parsley (chopped)
- 1 prize pepper
- 1 prize salt

PREPARATION

1. Divide the peppers lengthways, remove the stalk, wash and core and cut into thin strips.
2. Peel the onion and cut into small cubes or very thin strips.
3. Mix the paprika strips and chopped onion in a bowl with the vinegar, a little water, oil, the chopped parsley, pepper and salt.
4. Let the salad stand in the refrigerator for an hour.

PASTA SALAD

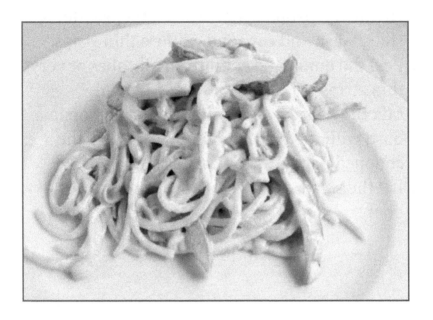

Servings:8

INGREDIENTS

- 1000 G Extra sausage, thinly sliced
- 250 G spaghetti
- 3 Pc Paprika (1 each yellow, red, green)
- 1 Pc Cucumber
- 200 G cheese
- 1 Can Corn
- 1 Glass Salad mayonnaise
- 4   Pc Cocktail tomatoes
- 1 prize pepper

- 1 prize salt
-

PREPARATION

1. For the pasta salad, cut the extra sausage into thin strips, as well as the cheese - also cut the remaining ingredients very thinly.
2. In the meantime, cook the spaghetti in salted water until al dente and cool.
3. Mix the cooled noodles with the remaining ingredients and season with salt and pepper as desired - let stand / steep in the refrigerator.

FETA AND MELON SALAD

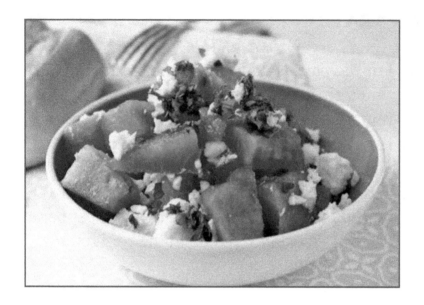

Servings:4

INGREDIENTS

- 0.5 Pc Watermelon
- 250 G Feta cubes
- 2 Pc Spring onion
- 15 Bl mint
- 4 Tbsp olive oil
- 1 priz salt

PREPARATION

1. Peel the melon, cut into cubes, remove the stones if necessary.
2. Chop the onion and mint into small pieces.
3. Then mix the melon, onion and mint with the olive oil and salt, finally add the cheese cubes and let them steep for a moment.

FRENCH DRESSING

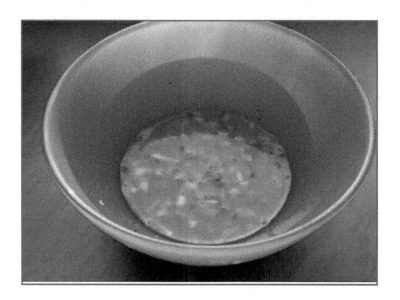

Servings:1

INGREDIENTS

- 1 Pc egg yolk
- 4 TL olive oil
- 1 TL mustard
- 0.5 Pc onion
- 0.5 Pc garlic
- 4 Tbsp Apple Cider Vinegar
- 1 TL honey
- 1 prize parsley
- 1 prize pepper

- 1 prize salt

PREPARATION

1. The egg yolk and the oil are mixed well with a whisk or hand blender until it is creamy.
2. Then the mustard is stirred into the French dressing.
3. Half the onion piece and the garlic are finely chopped and also added.
4. Finally, the French dressing is seasoned with a dash of apple cider vinegar, honey, pepper and salt.

TZATZIKI

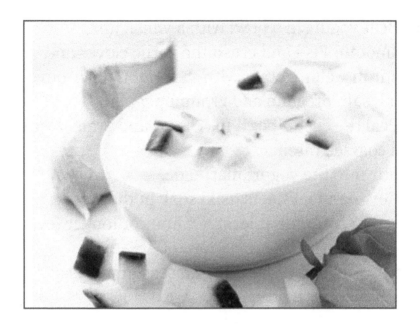

Servings:4

INGREDIENTS

- 3 Tbsp Yogurt fat
- 1 Pc Garlic cloves
- 1 Tbsp Lemon juice
- 3 Tbsp olive oil
- 0.5 TL salt
- 0.5 TL oregano
- 1 prize pepper
- 1 Pc Cucumber

PREPARATION

1. Beat yogurt in a bowl with a whisk until smooth. Peel and crush the garlic cloves and stir in well together with the lemon juice, olive oil, salt, oregano and ground pepper.
2. Peel the cucumber if necessary and grate it with a coarse grater.
3. Stir into the yogurt marinade.
4. Cover and let the tsatsiki soak in the refrigerator for at least 1/2 hour or longer (even overnight).
5. Stir well before serving and season with salt and pepper if necessary.

TOMATO AND AVOCADO SALAD

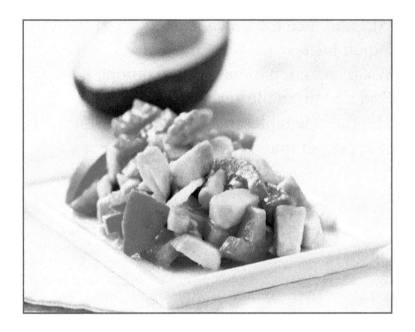

Servings:2

INGREDIENTS

- 2 Pc avocado
- 2 Pc tomatoes
- 4 Pc Spring onion
- 1 Pc Lemon (juice)
- 4 Pc Garlic cloves
- 5 Tbsp olive oil
- 1 prize pepper
- 1 prize salt

PREPARATION

1. Peel and dice the avocados and drizzle with lemon juice.
2. Wash and chop tomatoes and onions.
3. Peel and press the garlic.
4. Mix the vegetables in a bowl and season with salt, pepper and olive oil.

SHRIMP SALAD

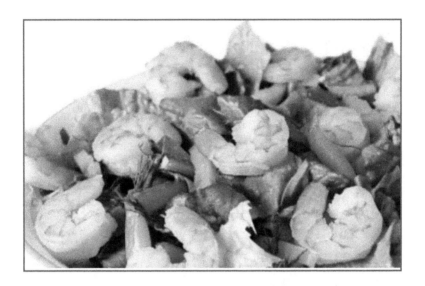

Servings:4

INGREDIENTS

- 4 Tbsp honey
- 2 Tbsp Lemon juice
- 1 prize pepper
- 1 kpf salad
- 4 Pc Carrots
- 4 Pc Peppers, green, red, yellow
- 500 G Shrimp

For the dressing
- 4 Tbsp honey
- 4 Tbsp Calvadossenf
- 2 Tbsp Lime juice
- 1 shot oil
-

PREPARATION

1. Drain the shrimp.
2. For the marinade, mix honey, lemon juice and pepper, brush the shrimp with it and let it steep for a few minutes.
3. Wash the lettuce, cut the vegetables into bite-sized pieces and place in a bowl.
4. Dressing: mix honey, calvadoss sauce and lime juice in a small bowl.
5. Finally, fold in a little oil.
6. Fry the shrimps in a pan with hot oil for a few minutes.
7. Spread the salad on a plate, pour the dressing over it and garnish with herbs and the shrimp.

POTATO SALAD WITH YOGURT

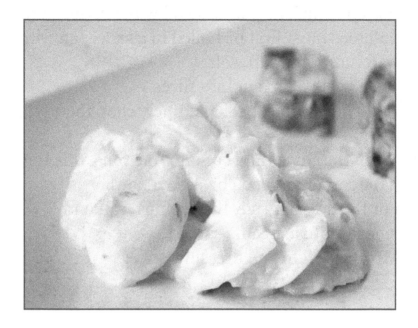

Servings:4

INGREDIENTS

- 4 Tbsp vinegar
- 200 ml yogurt
- 500 G Potatoes
- 1 TL salt
- 1 Federation chives
- 1 Pc onion

PREPARATION

1. For the delicious potato salad with yoghurt, the potatoes must first be boiled in a saucepan with water until they are soft.
2. Then peeled and cut into slices.
3. In the meantime, peel and finely chop the onion.
4. Wash the chives and cut into fine rolls. Mix the potatoes, onion and chives in a bowl.
5. For the dressing, stir the yoghurt, salt and vinegar into a creamy sauce.
6. Mix the potato and dressing well.

LENTIL SALAD WITH FETA

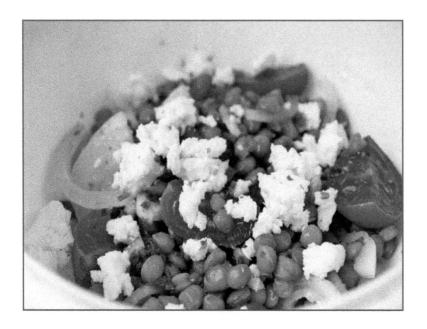

Servings:4

INGREDIENTS
- 3 Pc Spring onion
- 1 Can lenses
- 3 Pc tomatoes
- 250 G Feta
- 0.5 Federation thyme
- 4 Tbsp Balsamic vinegar
- 5 Tbsp olive oil
- 1 TL mustard
- 1 prize sugar

- 1 prize pepper
- 1 prize salt
-

PREPARATION

1. For the lentil salad with feta, drain the lentils well in a colander and then rinse them with cold water.
2. Wash, clean and chop the onion and tomatoes. Wash and finely chop the thyme in the same way. Cut the feta into cubes.
3. Now put everything in a bowl.
4. Mix a marinade from vinegar, mustard, oil, sugar, pepper and salt and pour over the salad. Mix carefully.

TUNA SALAD WITH RICE

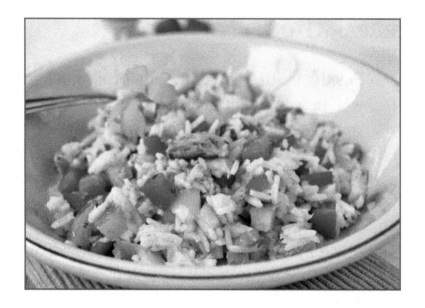

Servings:4

INGREDIENTS

- 250 G rice
- 2   Pc onion
- 2 Can tuna
- 1 Pc paprika
- 0.5 Pc cucumber
- 4 Tbsp vinegar
- 5 Tbsp oil
- 1 prize pepper
- 1 prize salt

PREPARATION

1. For the tuna salad with rice, first cook the rice according to the instructions on the packet, then drain it well in a sieve.
2. Likewise, let the tuna drain well in a colander.
3. Now peel and finely chop the onions. Wash the bell pepper and cucumber and cut into bite-sized pieces.
4. Put the vegetables, rice and tuna in a bowl.
5. Mix a dressing of oil, vinegar, salt and pepper in a bowl and marinate the salad with it.
6. Let the salad sit in the refrigerator for an hour and stir well before serving.

CELERY SALAD

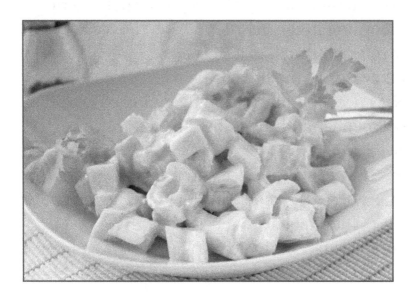

Servings: 2

INGREDIENTS

- 250 G Celeriac
- 1 Pc Apple
- 2 Tbsp Lemon juice
- 0.5 cups sour cream
- 1 prize sugar
- 1 prize pepper
- 1 prize salt

PREPARATION

1. Clean the celery, cut the stalks in half crosswise and cut lengthways into thin strips with a peeler.
2. Quarter and core the apple, cut into thin slices and mix with lemon juice.
3. Mix the sour cream with salt, sugar and pepper and mix well with the salad.

QUINOA SALAD WITH AVOCADO

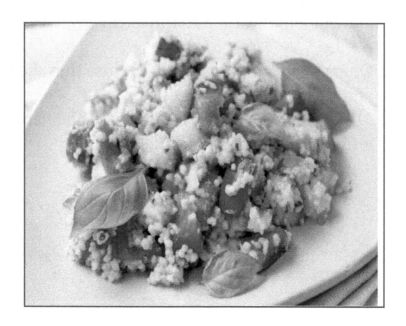

Servings:4

INGREDIENTS

- 1 Cup Quinoa
- 1 prize salt
- 1 prize pepper
- 1 Pc cucumber
- 100 ml water
- 1 Pc avocado
- 1 Federation parsley
- 1 shot olive oil

- 10 Pc Cocktail tomatoes

PREPARATION

1. First, the quinoa is covered with water in a saucepan and heated.
2. Let the quinoa simmer gently for about 15 minutes.
3. Meanwhile, wash the tomatoes and cucumber and cut into small pieces.
4. Remove the avocado from the skin and cut into small pieces.
5. When the quinoa is soft, it can be sieved and mixed with the tomato, cucumber, and avocado pieces.
6. Season with salt and pepper as needed, sprinkle with a little parsley and add a dash of oil.

MEDITERRANEAN PASTA SALAD WITH OLIVE DRESSING

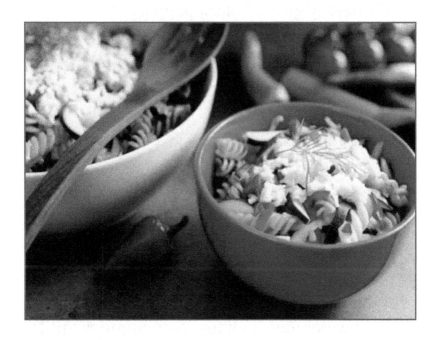

Servings:4

INGREDIENTS

- 250   G Spiral noodles
- 1 Pc Red pepper
- 1 Pc yellow or green peppers
- 1 Tbsp Sunflower oil
- 2 Tbsp olive oil
- 2   Pc Cloves of garlic, crushed
- 1 Pc Eggplant, diced
- 2   Pc Zuccini, cut into thick slices

- 2 Pc large tomatoes, peeled, without seeds
- 5 Tbsp flat-leaf parsley, chopped
- 1 TL freshly ground black pepper
- 150 G Feta cheese, crumbled
- for the olive dressing
- 2 Tbsp Balsamic vinegar
- 6 Pc Olives (black)
- 125 ml olive oil
- 1 prize pepper
- 1 prize salt
-

PREPARATION

1. Put the spiral pasta in a large saucepan with boiling water and cook for 10-12 minutes until al dente. Drain, spread out in a layer on a baking sheet and let dry.
2. Chill without the lid.
3. Halve the red and yellow peppers lengthways. Remove seeds and whites.
4. Cut the bell pepper into large pieces. Place with the cut side down under the preheated oven grill and brown until the skin blisters.
5. Let cool under a kitchen towel or in a transparent bag, peel off the skin and discard. Cut the paprika meat into thick strips.
6. Heat the sunflower and olive oil in a pan.

7. Add the garlic and aubergine and brown quickly, turning constantly. Remove from heat and pour into a large bowl. Steam the zucchini for 1-2 minutes until they are firm to the bite. Rinse under cold water, drain and add to the aubergines pieces.

8. Olive dressing: 6 large black olives, pitted, 125 ml olive oil, 2 tablespoons balsamic vinegar, salt, freshly ground black pepper. Chop the olives in the food processor. Slowly pour in olive oil and continue processing until a smooth mass is formed. Add vinegar, season with salt and freshly ground black pepper and stir until smooth.

9. Mix the pasta, bell pepper, aubergine, zucchini, tomatoes, parsley and pepper in a large bowl. Arrange on serving plates, pour the feta cheese over them and drizzle with the dressing.

CONCLUSIONS

A vegetarian diet focuses on eating vegetables. This includes dried fruits, vegetables, peas and beans, grains, seeds, and nuts. There is no single type of vegetarian diet.

Vegetarian diets continue to grow in popularity. The reasons for following a vegetarian diet are varied and include health benefits, such as reduced risk of heart disease, diabetes, and some types of cancer. However, some vegetarians consume too many processed foods, which can be high in calories, sugar, fat, and sodium, and may not consume enough fruits, vegetables, whole grains, and foods rich in calcium, missing out on the nutrients they provide.

However, with a little planning, a vegetarian diet can meet the needs of people of all ages, including children, adolescents, and pregnant or lactating women. The key is to be aware of your own nutritional needs so that you can plan a diet that meets them.

Vegan diets exclude beef, chicken, and fish, eggs, and dairy products, as well as foods that contain these products. Some people follow a semi-vegetarian diet (also called a flexitarian diet) which is primarily a plant-based diet but includes meat, dairy, eggs, chicken, and fish occasionally or in small amounts. How to plan a healthy vegetarian diet

To get the most out of a vegetarian diet, choose a good variety of healthy plant foods, such as whole fruits and vegetables, legumes, nuts, and whole grains. At the same time, cut down on less healthy options like sugar-sweetened beverages, fruit juices, and refined grains. If you need help, a registered dietitian can help you create a vegetarian plan that is right for you.

To get started

One way to transition to a vegetarian diet is to progressively reduce the meat in your diet while increasing your consumption of fruits and vegetables. Here are a couple of tips to help you get started:

Gradual transition. Increase the number of meatless meals you already enjoy each week, like spaghetti with tomato sauce or stir-fry vegetables. Find ways to include vegetables, such as spinach, kale, chard, and collards, in your daily meals.

Replacements. Take your favorite recipes and try them without meat. For example, make vegetarian chili by omitting the ground beef and adding an extra can of black beans. Or make fajitas using extra firm tofu instead of chicken. You will be surprised to find that many chain rings only require simple replacements.

Diversity. Buy or borrow vegetarian cookbooks. Visit ethnic restaurants to try new vegetarian recipes. The more variety your vegetarian diet has, the more likely you are to meet all of your nutritional needs.

The vegetarian diet, if it is prepared by choosing the foods appropriately and taking into account the guidelines and indications of the doctor or nutritionist, is able to provide the body with the nutrients it needs and to ensure the maintenance of a good state of health.

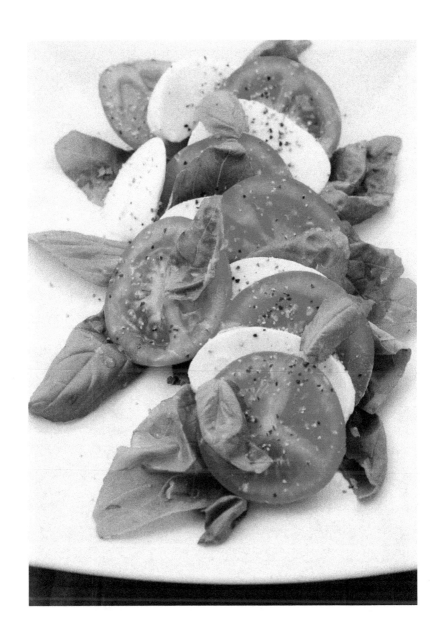

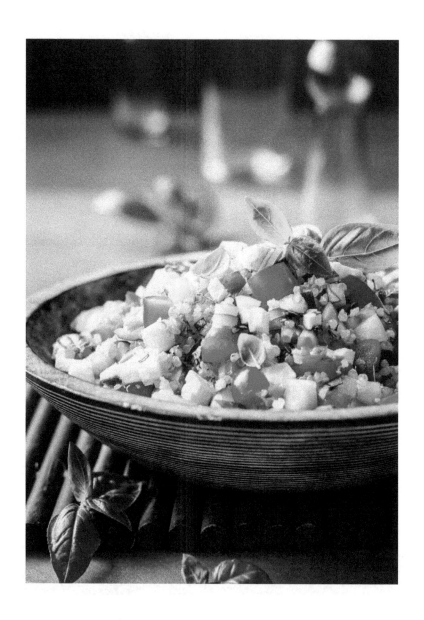

Lightning Source UK Ltd.
Milton Keynes UK
UKHW021256100521
383453UK00001B/104